Apple Cider Vinegar

The Amazing Guide on The Uses of ACV For Numerous Health Conditions, and How to Make it from Home

Dr. Michelle Ellen Gleen

This document is intended to provide accurate and dependable information about the subject and issues discussed. The publication is sold with the understanding that the publisher is not obligated to provide accounting, legally permissible, or otherwise qualified services. If legal or professional advice is required, a practicing member of the profession should be contacted.

From a Declaration of Principles that was unanimously accepted and approved by an American Bar Association Committee and a Publishers and Associations Committee.

The information contained herein is stated to be accurate and consistent, and any liability incurred as a result of inattention or otherwise as a result of the recipient reader's use or abuse of any policies, processes, or directions contained herein is sole and complete. Under no

ISBN: 978-1-63750-322-5

Free Bonus

Download my **"Keto Cookbook with 60+ Keto Recipes For Your Personal Enjoyment"** Ebook For **FREE!**

The **Keto Diet Cookbook** is a collection of **60+ delicious recipes** that are easy and fun to make in the comfort of your own home. It gives you the exact *recipes that you can use to prepare meals for any moment of the day, breakfast, lunch, dinner, and even dessert.*

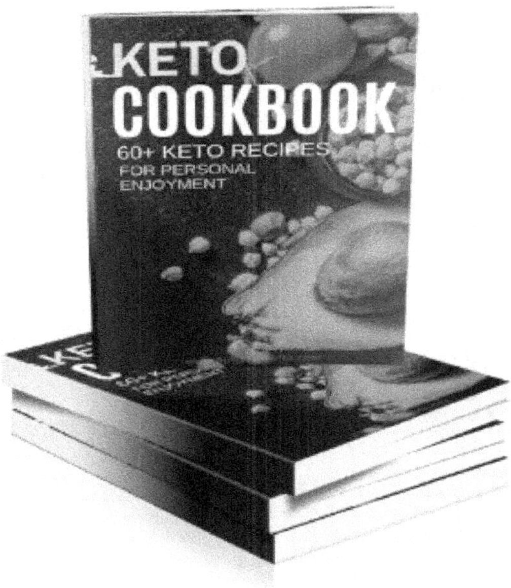

You don't need 5 different cookbooks with a ton of recipes to live a healthy and fun lifestyle. *You just need a good and efficient one and that is what the **Keto Diet Cookbook** is.*

Click the URL below to **Download the Book For FREE**, and also Subscribe for Free books, giveaways, and new releases by me. **https://mayobook.com/drmichelle**

My Books

Alkaline Diet: The Secret to Healthy Living with Alkaline Foods (Healthy Food Lifestyle)

The Alkaline Diet Cookbook: Your Guide to Eating More Alkaline Foods, and Less Acidic Foods For Healthy Living (Healthy Food Lifestyle)

Ketogenic Diet For Beginners: Your Complete Keto Guide and Cookbook with Low Carb, High-Fat Recipes For Living The Keto Lifestyle

Anti Inflammatory Diet Cookbook For Beginners: 3-Week Quick & Delicious Meal Plan with Easy Recipes to Heal The Immune Systems and Restore Overall Health

Apple Cider Vinegar: A Quick, Easy, and Affordable Guide to the Health Benefits, and Healing Power of Apple Cider Vinegar (ACV)

Apple Cider Vinegar: The Amazing Guide on The Uses of ACV For Numerous Health Conditions, and How to Make it from Home

Brain Cancer Awareness: How to Help Your Brain Fight Brain Cancer

Dr. Sebi Cookbook: Alkaline Diet Nutritional Guide with Sea moss, Medicinal Herbal Teas, Smoothies, Desserts, Mushroom, Salads, Soups & More, to Rejuvenate the Body with 100+ Recipes

Skin Tag Removal: How To Get Rid of Your Skin Tags in Simple Steps

Trigger Points: The New Self Treatment Guide to Pain Relief

Table of Contents

Introduction

Discover the miraculous properties of Apple Cider Vinegar (ACV) with this comprehensive guide, which gives you everything you need to know about the amazing healing properties of this simple, natural remedy.

If you're new to natural health and you don't know where to begin, then this is the guide for you. This book is packed with tons of useful information, and it will be a life-changer for those who read it.

Apple cider vinegar is a natural remedy that can do much more than simply give you a healthy glow. It can help fight cancer, ease digestion, lower cholesterol, prevent wrinkles, improve blood pressure, and even treat skin conditions. It is an ancient remedy used in Chinese medicine for hundreds of years. Today, it is being used by millions of people as a powerful natural remedy to treat a wide variety of health conditions. This guide explains why and how ACV is a powerful natural remedy for so many health conditions.

What is Apple Cider Vinegar?

Apple cider vinegar is made by fermenting apple juice with a culture of yeast and bacteria. It is one of the oldest known and most widely used home remedies. It was first made in the 13th century by monks in the Middle East. The name *"apple cider vinegar"* comes from the original process. It was made by fermenting fresh apple juice with a culture of bacteria and yeast.

If you're struggling with any health condition and you're not sure why you're suffering, you might want to give apple cider vinegar a try. Many people have found that it works very well to help cure a wide range of different health conditions. You've probably heard the term Apple Cider Vinegar used as a miracle product for countless health conditions and various skin care. But did you know that Apple Cider Vinegar is not only useful for healthy hair and skin care but can be used for numerous other health conditions?

There are countless natural uses of apple cider vinegar. Many experts say that drinking a cup of ACV mixed with water every morning is an excellent health hack. So, if you're looking to improve your health, consider adding one of these amazing uses for ACV into your daily routine.

Apple cider vinegar (ACV) is one of nature's most powerful natural health remedies. It has been used for centuries by herbalists and doctors as a cure for everything from arthritis to cancer. Many people use Apple Cider Vinegar (ACV) as a natural remedy for a wide variety of health conditions. It is one of the best home remedies for acidity, gas, indigestion, high cholesterol, and a variety of other problems.
This is not some fluff piece, but rather a concise, thorough, and well written guide to the uses of apple cider vinegar (ACV). There are only 4 major health conditions that ACV is purported to be helpful with. It goes into much detail about each condition, describing the studies and how it has been applied to each one.

And there is one thing that is very common in the research: vinegar has shown amazing results. Even if you're skeptical of vinegar's health benefits, you can't deny the fact that it has been used for hundreds of years. So if you want to get started, I recommend reading this book over and over. ACV is widely considered to be a probiotic, which means it is believed to be great for your gut health, which is essential for overall health.

According to the National Center for Complementary and Alternative Medicine (NCCAM), there are over 400 uses for apple cider vinegar (ACV). ACV is an ancient remedy with modern research revealing it can help you with everything from weight loss, heart disease, digestive disorders, and more. Here's the surprising thing—apple cider vinegar is one of the least expensive remedies available in the world and is often overlooked in the diet, but has amazing results for the healthiest skin. It is used extensively throughout Europe and Asia as a remedy for a variety of illnesses.

Apple cider vinegar is one of the best natural remedies for numerous health conditions. This versatile ingredient has been used for thousands of years. ACV is a rich source of many nutrients, including B vitamins, antioxidants, minerals, and enzymes. These nutrients contribute to healthy hair, skin, nails, digestion, and overall wellness. Plus, the acidic properties of ACV balance the pH of the blood, making it a great natural remedy for certain diseases like diabetes, arthritis, and cardiovascular disease.

This is a detailed guide with instructions for using apple cider vinegar (ACV) for a variety of health problems.

Chapter 1

Apple Cider Vinegar & Honey

You can mix honey with apple cider vinegar for variety of reasons.

There are a wide variety of fermentable carbohydrates that can be used to make vinegar. Apple cider vinegar is made by fermenting apple juice twice with yeast as a basis. Acetic acid is the primary constituent, which is why it has a sour taste.

If you'd like, you may think of honey as a sticky, delicious material made by bees that is stored in honeycombs. Fructose and glucose are the two main sugars in honey, with trace amounts of pollen, minerals, and antioxidants also present. As the sweetness of honey helps to soften vinegar's puckery taste, many consider apple cider vinegar and honey a delicious pairing.

There are numerous health benefits to taking this tonic. As a result, it's hard to say what the specific effects of the combination will be because both substances have been studied on their own.

In natural medicine, both apple cider vinegar and honey can be consumed alone or in combination. Little research has looked into the medical implications of mixing these two, though.

ACV and Honey's Health Benefits

Because of the alleged health benefits, many individuals combine apple cider vinegar with honey.

Help relieve the symptoms of seasonal allergies and common cold

The antibacterial properties of honey and apple cider vinegar have been long debated. Because honey includes trace amounts of pollen and plant components, it has long been used to treat seasonal allergies. According to several studies, it may help alleviate the symptoms of allergic rhinitis, also known as hay fever.

Adding apple cider vinegar to honey has yet to be determined. Coughing, for example, may be eased by taking the mixture. As a bonus, apple cider vinegar contains probiotics thanks to its fermentation process. Digestive and immune-boosting bacteria are found in foods like *yogurt and sauerkraut.*

Taking acetic acid can help you lose weight

Apple cider vinegar's acetic acid is still being explored as a weight-loss aid.

Over the course of a 12-week study of 144 obese people, those who drank 17 ounces of apple cider vinegar diluted with 2 tablespoons (30 ml) of vinegar each day lost the greatest amount of weight and had the least amount of excess fat. Because it slows the rate at which nutrients are taken into the bloodstream, apple cider vinegar has been demonstrated to keep you feeling satisfied longer, which could help you shed pounds.

Still, note that honey is high in calories and sugar, and should be drunk in moderation when combined with vinegar.

Many studies have looked at the benefits of apple cider vinegar and honey separately, but few have looked at the effects of combining them.

It improves cardiovascular health

As a result of the chlorogenic acid in vinegar, you may be able to reduce your risk of heart disease. A study done on rats found that honey can lower high blood pressure, which is another risk factor for heart disease.

Along with decreasing LDL cholesterol oxidation, polyphenol antioxidants also help lower the risk of heart disease by increasing blood flow and dissolving blood clots. Despite this, additional work in this area is needed. Aside from reducing inflammation and lowering the risk of arterial plaque buildup, apple cider vinegar may also safeguard your heart health. However, further human research is needed to investigate this putative benefit. Apple cider vinegar's health benefits are largely unexplored, while honey's are well-documented. Vinegar is thought to help with weight loss, and both vinegar and apple cider vinegar are thought to improve heart health and relieve colds and seasonal allergies.

Alleviate heart diseases

Apple cider vinegar's high acidity may exacerbate stomach reflux, but some people have stated that it has helped alleviate their symptoms. Due to the lack of conclusive data, pay attention to your body's signals instead. In addition, apple cider vinegar's acidity has been shown to erode dental enamel, which makes it more likely that teeth will get cavities.

Because of this, vinegar shouldn't be diluted with filtered water and rinsed from the mouth with water after consumption. The results of mixing it with honey must be studied further. Studies reveal that honey can help prevent gingivitis, cavities, and bad breath as well.

The potential impact on blood sugar levels and triglyceride levels

A study that looked at the identical combo of grape vinegar and honey found that it had some negative impacts on health. Some participants in the four-week study found that their insulin resistance increased slightly when they drank 8.5 oz of water mixed with 4 tsp of grape vinegar, honey, and numerous mints for flavor each day.

Type 2 diabetes is linked to insulin resistance.

The HDL (very good) cholesterol, which has been shown to protect the heart, also fell towards the end of the study. HDL (bad) cholesterol is linked to cardiovascular disease. Remember that it was simply a small and brief experiment. These findings need to be verified by other studies. Honey and apple cider vinegar, rather than grape vinegar, should be studied in a documented report.

Alkalinity-enhancing properties

From the most acidic to the most alkaline states, the pH scale measures acidity and alkalinity. Some people say alkaline foods and supplements such as applesauce and honey may help prevent cancer and osteoporosis, although the evidence is mixed.

It's important to keep your blood pH level between 7.35 and 7.45 because it's critical to your body's overall health and function. Blood pH can be dangerous if it slips outside of this range. Blood alkalinity is not significantly affected by foods or supplements, including different kinds of apple cider vinegar and honey. Your urine's pH level is only affected by what you eat. Whether or not apple cider vinegar can change your body's acid-base balance over time has yet to be researched.

Apple cider vinegar, according to some, can alkalize your body and lower your risk of disease. Diets and supplements only change the pH of your urine, but your body takes care of your blood pH levels.

Sugar content

Depending on how much honey you use, your mixture will contain a lot of sugar. In order to maintain a healthy lifestyle, it is imperative that you minimize the amount of added sugar in your diet. There is a larger risk of conditions, including heart disease and obesity, if you consume a lot of added sugar, particularly from sweetened beverages.

Despite the fact that a tiny amount of honey can match a healthy diet and may provide health benefits, you should be thankful in moderation. It is possible that drinking apple cider vinegar and honey can have negative effects on oral and digestive health. The medical effects and dangers of the combo need to be studied further.

ACV's Best Uses

Drenched in 8 ounces of lukewarm to warm water, a relaxing tonic made from 1 tablespoon (15ml) of apple cider vinegar and 2 teaspoons (21 gms) of honey is used as a night or morning remedy in natural medicine. For additional flavor, try adding a pinch of cayenne pepper, fresh mint, or lemon juice to this steaming concoction. One hour before you go to sleep is the best time to drink it if you suffer from gastric reflux or heartburn.

It's also a good idea to use both apple cider vinegar and honey in a cooking environment. As a base for salad dressings, marinades, and brines for pickling vegetables, they are excellent. The safety of mixing apple cider vinegar with honey, on the other hand, has not been evaluated in tiny children. Before using this mixture as a home cure, you should speak with your child's pediatrician.

Due to the danger of botulism, a condition caused by bacteria that is rare but can be fatal, honey and apple cider vinegar should not be given to children under the age of one year due to the danger of botulism. Many people could benefit from using apple cider vinegar and honey on a regular basis. Dilute the mixture in hot water and take it as a hot tonic before going to bed or when you first get up. To make salads, marinate meats, and pickle vegetables, you can find everything in your kitchen.

In natural medicine, it's common to find both apple cider vinegar and honey.

Warm water is usually added to dilute the concoction, and it is then consumed before going to bed or right after waking up. It's claimed to aid in weight loss, reduce allergies, and enhance blood pressure. In most studies, however, the effects of each substance are studied independently. It's a pleasant and soothing drink to enjoy at the beginning or end of the day, but little is known about its potential medical benefits.

Chapter 2

How to Make Apple Cider Vinegar from Home

For a long time, home winemakers relied on simple fermentation techniques. Vinegar, on the other hand, is a more formal French term meaning "sour wine." If you can make wine at home, you should be able to get apple cider vinegar in your house. It takes a little while to do this work. But the intricacies of how it's done are a real treat. Making apple cider vinegar at home isn't as difficult as you would think. Using organic apples to make cider is generally a good idea. Wash and quarter the apples (there are around ten of them). Rest these slices at room temperature before serving. It goes without saying that they will turn brown. Fill a glass jar halfway with water and add the brown apples. Slices should be submerged in enough water to drown them.

Now, simply place a cheesecloth over the jar and secure it with a rubber band. To allow the apples, which have been soaked in regular water, to breathe oxygen, you do not need to knot or secure them. Now, find a warm spot in your house and just install the entire equipment there. At the very least, give this jar six months to rest. Make sure to give it a good stir once a week at the very least. Consider this jar to be empty after six months. At the jar's rim, you'll see a layer of scum accumulating.

This is what happens when bacteria cause apple fermentation. When you shake a few soaps into a bucket of water, the layer will resemble the bubbles you find in the water.

The liquid will be filtered next. Place the apple jar in a larger one and cover it with cheesecloth. This time, secure the cheesecloth firmly. It's as simple as swiping the smaller container over the larger one. This will allow the liquid to flow into the second container. Allow all of the liquid to be transferred to the larger container.

For now, allow the fresh jar of liquid to sit in a warm place. For at least a month, it won't be touched. Waiting for the gorgeous amber-colored apple cider vinegar should be worth it. You may use it in numerous home remedies.

There are various advantages to making your own apple cider vinegar. They not only produce superior outcomes, but because they are purer, they pose a lower danger of side effects. Because you were the one who acquired it, the cleanliness and hygiene of the entire process will be guaranteed to you. Of course, the first few times will be a real test of your endurance. In the end, you'll get the satisfaction of making these unique foods at home and reaping the health benefits.

Precautions

In terms of treating a wide range of diseases, there is no question that apple cider vinegar is superior. However, we must also make sure that the product is ingested in the appropriate quantities. They don't have any negative health consequences or concerns. There is a danger, however, of overdoing it. Apple cider vinegar is a good example of this.

Chapter 3

ACV Miracle Healing Uses

"An apple a day keeps the doctor away" is a well-known adage among many people. They've got common sense. It is one of God's most nutritious foods. Acquiring potassium for the soft tissues in the body as calcium does for the bones and hard tissue is surely a good thing to do with apples. As an *"artery softener,"* potassium helps keep the blood vessels in the body flexible and resilient.

It is an antidote to harmful bacteria and viruses. *"An apple a day keeps the doctor away,"* which is, in fact, a sound, down-to-earth natural medicine for healthy, long-term health. Yes!! The apple is a time-honored favorite. When it comes to fruit, it is one of the oldest things that humans have ever eaten. The fruit from your Garden of Eden has played a significant role in shaping our future. For a long time, people have been consuming applications. If you don't eat apples, you'll never be as healthy as someone who does. Potassium is a crucial mineral in the apple's nutritional constellation; without it, there would be no life! Apples are tasty fruits that many people enjoy devouring. This deficiency can be found not just in the body's cells but also across the entire organism. Look around and see how many people you can find that exude an aura of health.

Your physical well-being is your greatest asset.

Potassium Deficiency Problems

There are millions of people who are suffering from potassium insufficiency because of modern civilization's reliance on commercially prepared meals. Neither your skin nor your muscles look good. The body's skeletal framework will not be firmly held in place by the flesh. The skin on the face and neck is wrinkled and wrinkly. One telltale indication is the appearance of sagging, drooping skin around the eyes. The drooping eyelids progress as the potassium deficit worsens. Instead of wide-open eyes, people will start looking for tiny openings in them. In order to improve hooded eyelids, which roll down and rest around the eyelashes and cause fatigue and headaches, many people have considered having eyelid surgery. As a result, it's not uncommon for an insurance company to cover any necessary corrective surgery recommended by an eye specialist as a result of this. It's a simple in-and-out process.

The best option is to choose a board-certified surgeon. People mistakenly attribute their sagging eyelids, wrinkles, and lack of muscular tone to their age. However, potassium is essential for the formation and maintenance of youthful and healthy tissues! A senile appearance will quickly set in if the recommended daily potassium intake is not met. A potassium shortage and an unhealthy lifestyle are usually to blame for this premature aging.

The same rules apply to your vegetable and flower gardens. Potassium is necessary for the development of chemicals that give the stems of plants stiffness and boost their resistance to certain plant diseases. It is possible that potassium can transform seeds into plants and flowers through a process of gradual development. When plants lack potassium, they stop growing. If the potassium shortage is not remedied, the plant gradually deteriorates, turning yellow and eventually dying!

A potassium deficit has the same effect on both animals and humans. The cells slowly degenerate until they die and are no longer able to sustain life.

Body Cleansing with Apple Cider Vinegar

Time changes and you aren't able to carry out the important tasks in your life because you are depleted of human go power and vital force! It's time to clear out the toxic waste that's clogging your organs of elimination and draining your energy reserves! This ACV process flushes out the waste that has been split. Keep in mind that your colon, lungs, epidermis, and kidneys are all critical organs for waste removal. This group could end up being your loyal employees! In order to rid themselves of toxins, they put in a lot of effort every day. The ACV drink provides assistance for these emetic organs, which are frequently in need. You'll learn more about the ACV daily routine as you continue reading.

ACV can also be mixed into a salt-free tomato or fresh vegetable juice (such as carrots and greens) and consumed daily in between meals, using 1 teaspoon per 6 ounces of liquid.

Be sure to fast one day a week for cleaning and to follow the way of life described in this chapter to the letter.

Headaches cured with Apple Cider Vinegar

Numerous bodily parts have been implicated as causes of headaches, according to those who suffer from them. Allergies and sinusitis are very common causes of headaches, as are eyestrain, nerve damage, and digestive issues. Headaches can be divided into two categories: acute and chronic. It is possible that certain types of chronic headaches are brought on by a buildup of toxins and other illnesses. A headache serves as a warning sign to the normal individual that the body's deterioration is far from over. As the huge, red-flashing warning signal from Mother Nature, pain and headaches must be taken seriously. Anywhere in the body could have issues. The liver, gallbladder, kidneys, bowel, or other organs of the body may be affected.

Sensitive sinus, allergy, or mucus problems, for example, could be linked to or cause this. Avoid these meals that cause headaches:

- Foods loaded with additives and chemicals
- Foods that contain caffeine
- salty, sweet, or wheat-based foodstuffs.

- MSG, sulfites, and other additives
- Dairy products, particularly cheese, are a good source of calcium.
- "alcohol," "beer," and "wine"

Emotional headaches are the second type! Anxiety or any other psychological or emotional issues are to blame for this. You can get into a lot of emotional trouble if you live your life with people in a way that causes you to feel fear, jealousy, envy, hatred, greed, self-pity, or self-indulgence. If you let your emotions get the better of you, you may get a dull, throbbing headache. The worst headache is a migraine, which causes the patient to feel as if their skull is splintering apart.

Research on a wide range of headaches has shown that when the body causes a headache, it produces alkaline urine rather than acidic. Emotions can cause the kidneys to become inflamed, causing the body to become out of whack. By assisting the kidneys in regenerating urine with the proper acidity (an average pH of 6.4), ACV's malic acid quickly relieves headaches. ACV in vaporized form may also provide headache relief.

Pour 2 Tbsps of ACV and 2 cups of filtered water into a vaporizer or small pan. Bring the water to a boil.Turn off the heat, place a towel over the steam, and lean over it while inhaling five slow, deep breaths of the ACV steam vapors as they rise.

As a last resort, you can also apply hot and cold vinegar compresses to the forehead and neck area, as well as perform some shoulder/neck rolls and massage the head and shoulders.

Use 500 mg of bromelain for pain relief; it works like aspirin without the side effects or dangerous side effects. Many chronic headache sufferers have told us that this technique has given them a new lease of life.

These steps, along with a healthy lifestyle, should allow you to avoid the use of over-the-counter pain relievers and headache cures altogether.

ACV Enhances a Weight-Loss Plan

Every year, millions of individuals begin diets for a variety of reasons: a new year's resolve, a wedding, prepping for bikini season, or any number of other reasons. However, many of the fat loss products, portions, and strategies fail to deliver, leaving people who paid attention misled but still trying to lose those unwanted pounds. To lose weight and keep it off, the most successful diet and exercise regimens call for a healthy diet and regular exercise, both of which apple cider vinegar can help with.

Making use of ACV as part of your weight loss regimen is simple and effective.

Combine the following to get a daily dose:

- Drinking water in the amount of one cup
- 1-teaspoon of ACV
- 1 teaspoon lemon juice

To reap the benefits of the concoction's many health benefits, drink it at least five times a day before meals.

The following are commonly cited as four additional roadblocks to successfully losing weight and keeping it off:

- Being unable to control one's hunger or cravings
- To eat until one is full
- A lack of dynamism
- An inability to burn calories quickly

Those obstacles can be addressed because of the ACV's naturally occurring components. You'll learn even more about how to utilize ACV for weight loss as you continue reading.

Rapid Metabolic Rates

Right? Is this something that only "slim" people have? Wrong!

Despite the fact that genetics has a significant influence on metabolism, everyone has the ability to increase their metabolic rate through natural means. Try these energizing recipes for ACV.

To mix a drink, combine the following ingredients in the following order:

- A cup of green tea with herbs.
- 2 tablespoons apple cider vinegar.
- About a teaspoon of lemon juice.
- 1 teaspoon ground cayenne pepper.

Drink this metabolism-enhancing tonic 30 minutes before each meal to get the most benefit.

Caffeinated drinks, cayenne pepper, and a variety of vitamins and minerals in lemon juice and ACV all work together to boost metabolism, burn fat, and give you more energy.

In addition, you can speed up your metabolism in a couple of weeks by making the following little lifestyle adjustments:

Increase your fat-burning muscle mass by implementing a strength-training regimen. 4-6 days a week, do 30 minutes of cardiovascular exercise, and eat smaller meals more regularly.

It inhibits your eating habits

While on a diet, have you ever looked in the fridge for something to satisfy your hunger pangs? In spite of your best efforts to eat healthily and drink enough water, you'll still feel hungry and have an insatiable hunger, which can quickly lead to a diet derailment. Choose apple cider vinegar instead of giving in to temptation or enduring hunger and deprivation symptoms. This is a healthy choice.

To mix a drink, combine the following ingredients in the following order:

- 2 mugs of plain water.
- 1-teaspoon of ACV

To do this, stir well and sip every day.

Acidity levels in the stomach are normalized by the enzymes and acetic acid in ACV, resulting in less hunger and a smaller appetite. Other explanations for why ACV aids in appetite regulation will be presented. It's possible that the acetic acid in ACV slows down the glycemic index of foods, allowing for a longer sensation of satiety after meals and lessening the desire to snack. Another possibility is that the pectin in ACV expands when it comes into contact with water or other liquids, thereby decreasing one's appetite. Whatever the mechanism, it's possible! The best aspect about this tonic is that it's simple to make and quite portable, making it an easy substitute for the meals you'd consume and regret later.

Remind yourself to use your ACV appetite suppressant by placing a sticky note or index card on your refrigerator or cabinet where your selected craving foods are kept. You'll see the reminder every time you reach for something that isn't on your diet-friendly list.

Fasting Aids

Fasting is perhaps the oldest and most tried-and-true remedy for ridding your body of toxins and giving yourself a "break" from an overindulgent diet. In just a few days, you can start a new way of eating clean and living better by using a simple and quick ACV solution. Even if you usually drink alcohol, eat fattening foods, or have an unhealthy way of eating and drinking, you can start this new way of eating and drinking in just a few days.

When it comes to an easy meal, some people look forward to feeling revived and refreshed, while others are afraid of starving. Contemplate ACV *"fasting"* if you're hesitant to even consider it. It isn't like many other options in that you can still eat with the quick. *"Pioneer"* apple cider vinegar manufacturer and promoter, Paul C. Bragg. Throughout his life, he relied on his product to help him keep his health insurance, vitality, and ability to fend off sickness. It was his recommendation to use his product (Bragg's organic unfiltered ACV) in a tonic meant to flush out the device's waste while also adhering to a diet consisting solely of whole foods such as fruits and vegetables, nuts and seeds, and nut milks. With ACV, fruits, and vegetables flushed through the device, it helps the body's processes remove waste that has built up. By "keeping things moving" throughout this cleanse, your body will adapt naturally to a diet of whole, nutritious food.

Combine the following ingredients to make Bragg's tonic:

- 1 cup of regular water
- ACV, 1 teaspoon (or start with ½ teaspoons and work your way up to at least 1 teaspoon).
- One-half teaspoon of lemon juice.

For 7 to 10 days, eat 3-5 times a day.

Toxins are removed from the liver

Few people are aware of the liver's functions. Bile is secreted by the liver, which aids digestion. However, the liver's tasks go well beyond that! protecting and promoting one's health and vitality by:

- In order to efficiently break down fats, the body must remove waste and waste from the blood by making proteins and storing carbohydrates and other important nutrients.

Maintaining good health and well-being means keeping the liver free of harmful substances that make it less able to work properly.

You can maintain optimal liver function by following a diet plan and leading a lifestyle that places less strain on the liver:

- In order to stay healthy, eat a lot of fruits, vegetables, nuts, and seeds.
- Consume only a small amount of alcohol.
- Make sure you drink enough water and other liquids that are readily available (preferably water).
- If you don't need it, don't use it! (prescription and otherwise).

Apple cider vinegar is an ideal liver detoxification remedy because of the vitamins, nutrients, and enzymes it contains, all of which help to keep the pH level in check.

To prepare a liver-cleansing beverage, combine:

- Drinking water in the amount of one cup
- 1–2 tbsp. ACV
- ½ tsp. of unprocessed honey

Drink at least three times per day.

Cleaning of the gallbladder

Gallstones, which are waste products from the liver, can be eliminated from the body through the gallbladder's production of bile. The gallbladder and liver work in tandem to keep the body's pH balanced and remove toxins that are harmful to health. Maintaining the organ's fitness is critical to overall health, which is why an apple cider vinegar flush of the gallbladder is recommended. You'll benefit from twice-yearly gallbladder cleanses if you follow these guidelines.

Prepare it by mixing the following ingredients:

- 1 cup of regular water
- half tbsp. ACV
- 2 tbsp. of honey (organic, unfiltered).

Consume it twice a year, if possible.

Preventing gallstones is another benefit of a gallbladder cleaning like this. People with gallstones often don't show any symptoms, although some suffer from agonizing agony as a result of gallstones.

These are the most common causes of gallstones:

i. When the liver makes too much cholesterol, it crystallizes in the gallbladder and forms gallstones when there isn't enough bile to break it down.

ii. When the bile has a high concentration of bilirubin (the result of the chemical breakdown of red blood cells),
iii. Thirdly, there is a liver disease known as cirrhosis, which results in high levels of bilirubin being produced by the liver.
iv. Because of this, bile builds up in the gallbladder and eventually crystallizes into gallstones, which can be painful to pass through.

Gallstones can impede the flow of bile out of the gallbladder, resulting in excruciating agony. The ACV cleanse is a terrific way to help you avoid these problems all together.

Heartburn is relieved

The sheer number of people who suffer from heartburn could make finding a remedy difficult. Pre-and post-meal pills, drinks, and other simple ways are all that's needed to alleviate the burden. Get rid of those other options and try apple cider vinegar, which has been used for a long time to treat heartburn. Competitors assert that the claim may be unsupported by science, but many people claim it works miracles. What are the last things you'd consider letting go of? Nothing. Give the natural option a chance.

To mix a cocktail, combine the following ingredients in the following order:

- Drinking water in the amount of one cup
- 1 teaspoon of apple cider vinegar
- 1 teaspoon of honey.

Once heartburn has subsided, drink every 30 minutes to reap the benefits of this remedy.

The real cause of heartburn may be an imbalance of stomach acids, which may be due to these factors:

- A deficiency in fat breakdown efficiency on your part.
- response to a nutrient-deficient diet that is insufficient.
- It looks as though your stomach is always battling with food rather than simply accepting it.

Apple cider vinegar may be important because of the acetic acid that comes from the fermentation of the apples used to make it.

Even though it sounds counterintuitive that adding acid will help with heartburn, the naturally occurring acetic acid in ACV pales in comparison to the hydrochloric acid produced in the stomach. The buffering effect helps to reduce and end heartburn by lowering the stomach's acidity back to a more normal level.

It prevents bloating and gas

Excessive flatulence is one of the most humiliating things a person may experience. There are thousands of over-the-counter remedies for excessive gas and flatulence that are both embarrassing, uncomfortable, and difficult to deal with. However, pills and drinks that promise to reduce the incidence of gas may be effective, but they often contain a plethora of chemicals and ingredients that you can't even pronounce. Excess gas can be caused by a wide range of medical conditions, but many people who suffer from bloating and gas on a regular basis blame processed foods. Unhealthy diets do a lot of damage to the digestive system, which causes gas to build up as a result.

Diets rich in fiber roughage, such as cruciferous vegetables (broccoli, cauliflower, etc.), can cause gas buildup and flatulence in people who consume too much of it regularly. No matter what the source may be, ACV can assist in eliminating gas. Flatulence can be reduced by eating a diet rich in complete foods that soothe gas-producing illnesses, including honey, fennel, ginger, and flaxseed, as well as all-natural ACV tonics that treat gas. Gas production and flatulence are cut down by ACV's active acids and enzymes, which neutralize the parts and processes that make gas.

To make a tonic for gas, combine the following ingredients:

- 1 cup of regular water
- 1 teaspoon honey
- 1 teaspoon of peppermint extract (optional)
- half teaspoon of cinnamon
- 1 tablespoon of ACV

Drink every day.

Reduce the severity of nausea and vomiting by lowering the temperature

Stomachaches can be the result of a variety of factors, ranging from psychological stress and unhealthy lifestyle choices to bad habits and prolonged exposure to unhealthy irritants. Acute stomach pain may occur from time to time, or you may be plagued by less severe but longer-lasting symptoms. There is no one-size-fits-all approach to dealing with stomachaches; it's best to focus on the root cause of your discomfort. Preventing and treating stomachaches can be as simple as making sure your entire digestive system, from your saliva to your colon, is working properly. ACV fights stomachaches from the inside out by balancing the pH in the entire digestive tract. ACV can help your body get rid of possible illnesses or invaders that could make you sick or make you more uncomfortable by killing bacteria, viruses, and other harmful things.

To make a drink, combine the following ingredients in the following order:

- Drinking water in the amount of one cup
- 1 teaspoon apple cider vinegar

Stomachaches can be relieved by drinking this solution for 30 minutes at a time.

Ease morning sickness during pregnancy

Only a mother can truly appreciate the many facets of pregnancy. Pregnancy miracles like watching your tummy develop or feeling your first kick can be exhilarating and delightful during pregnancy. Pregnancy, however, has its share of drawbacks, such as nausea, vomiting, and stomach cramps. This jittery sensation, also known as *"morning sickness,"* can occur at any time of day or night and can range in severity from mild to severe.Some women choose to *"ride out"* their morning sickness because of the different degrees of discomfort. Some people seek relief from their symptoms by taking prescription medications. Morning sickness is as individual as the person who experiences it, but apple cider vinegar is an all-natural therapy that may help soothe or treat the symptoms of morning sickness.

Combine the following ingredients to make a morning sickness remedy:

- 1 cup of plain water.
- ½ to at least one 1 tablespoon of ACV
- ½ peeled ginger juice

Take a sip of the concoction every hour for around an hour to get some relief.

The following minerals and vitamins are included in ACV and may assist both the mother and the fetus during pregnancy:

- Vitamins A, B, C, and E are included in this category.
- The potassium-magnesium-iron group of minerals
- easier-to-digest fiber and probiotics.

Pregnant women benefit the following tremendously from the combination of these nutrients:

- Keep their bodies' pH levels in check.
- Helps digestion by neutralizing digestive enzymes.

- Constipation and diarrhea are two other factors that might contribute to morning sickness and therefore they help in relieving them.

Constipation is eased with the use of this remedy

Constipation is, without a doubt, a debilitating illness of the digestive system. You may have a persistent impression that you need to go forward but are unable to do so. Your stomach hurts, your breath stinks (constipation is often accompanied by bad breath!), and you're plagued with gas and bloating. But you don't give up hope. Adding insult to injury is the fact that this position can last more than a week at a time. Regular pee-peeers may start to feel the excruciating pain of constipation a few hours after they have their regular pee-pee.

A wide variety of treatments can be found in the medicine cabinets of your local drugstore. However, many of these products are laden with chemicals that might have harmful side effects or even produce explosive repercussions. If you want a more natural substitute for various sorts of constipation alleviation, look no further than your favorite bottle of apple cider vinegar.

Constipation can be alleviated by ingesting apple cider vinegar (ACV), which contains pectin, iron, acetic acid, and fiber, which forms a goo-like fibrous supplement in the digestive system and aids in the movement of stool. Many people can go to the bathroom in about an hour or two, and they don't have to deal with any extreme side effects. This is like a softer, fuller stool form.
To feel better right away, simply combine the following:

- 1 tablespoon of ACV
- A cup of water

Drink the mixture over the course of 30 minutes.

Try the following combination of therapies to prevent the problem from reoccurring:

- Take this mixture three times a day.
- Drink a lot more water than usual.
- Caffeinated drinks should be avoided at all costs.
- Nuts and seeds are a good source of natural fiber and should be eaten in their whole form whenever possible.

Get Rid of Your Diarrhea

Diarrhea always seems to strike at the most inconvenient times. It doesn't matter if you're in your own home or at a black-tie gala; this debilitating ailment will always be with you. Because diarrhea could be the body's way of dealing with an unwanted component of the digestive system, it is recognized as a signal rather than a problem. If the irritant is a deep-fried food that isn't being properly digested, a virus attempting to attack the condition's fighting capability, or an even more extreme case of parasites, diarrhea could be the body's natural method of quickly purging the irritant from your own body and protecting one's health and vitality. Over-the-counter diarrhea medications designed to stop you from going aren't the proper remedy because diarrhea rids the body of the severe irritant. To get rid of an irritant, you would have to take a diarrhea-curing solution. Instead, the irritant would clog your digestive system and cause problems for the rest of your life.

If you get constipation as a side effect of your medication, you've just made a bad situation worse. Pectin, iron, and acetic acid are all components of apple cider vinegar that aid in the natural resolution of diarrhea. As a lubricant in the digestive system, it also adds bulk to the stool. Regardless of what happens, this is not a matter of miracles! Within thirty minutes, ACV moves waste through your body in a way that is more comfortable than anything you've ever had before.

To prepare a drink to resolve diarrhea, combine:

- A cup of hot water
- 1-2 tablespoon of apple cider vinegar

For a quarter of an hour, sip on the concoction. This remedy can be taken as many times as necessary until the diarrhea stops, up to a maximum of three times an hour.

Preventing Bacterial Cystitis (UTI)

The medical phrase "urinary tract infection," or UTI, can be used interchangeably with the term "bacterial cystitis." Bacteria are the most common cause of cystitis, which is commonly referred to as bladder inflammation. Interstitial cystitis is frequently the deciding factor in determining whether or not the infection is due to bacteria. It's not just women who are at risk for bacterial cystitis; men and children can also be affected. Women are more likely to get parasites because their urethras are shorter, which makes them more vulnerable to the bugs.

Tingling is the first sign of trouble, but as the condition worsens, the sufferer may have the urge to urinate more frequently, with or without urine coming out. Other symptoms may include discomfort and burning when urinating. Antibiotics are the most common treatment for bacterial cystitis, which is caused by a bacterial infection in the bladder. It is possible to prevent and ameliorate the issue by using natural methods.

Apple cider vinegar, which is rich in vitamins and minerals, is an excellent preventative alternative for bacterial cystitis since it flushes the body of poisons just like the parasites that contribute to this discomfort. There are two methods you can use to accomplish this:
To mix a drink, combine the following ingredients in the following order:

- Drinking water in the amount of one cup
- 1 tablespoon of apple cider vinegar

Drink water every day.

Before starting an ACV regimen, most women reported experiencing fewer cases of bacterial cystitis as well as less severe symptoms if the concoction was taken as prescribed.

Alternatively, you may want to experiment with this bathing technique:

In the tub, combine the following ingredients:

- A cup of apple cider vinegar (ACV)
- Fill the tub with warm water and relax!

Take a 30-minute bath.

By destroying germs in the urethra, this wash relieves symptoms.

Limits Interstitial Cystitis

In contrast to bacterial cystitis, interstitial cystitis is a long-term disorder characterized by inflammation of the bladder's submucosal and muscular layers rather than the bladder itself. Interstitial cystitis, also known as bladder pain syndrome (BPS), can manifest as a variety of unpleasant symptoms, including blood in the urine, acute pelvic discomfort, and the sudden need to urinate 60 times a day, whether or not any urine is actually evacuated. The fact that there is no known cause or solution for this illness is perhaps the most ominous aspect of it. It's not clear if it's a congenital disability, caused by vascular disease, or made worse by allergies.

Because there is no known therapy for this ailment, many people who have it are left to suffer in silence or, in the worst-case scenario, have their bladders surgically removed. Some people with interstitial cystitis choose to take preventative steps that they can do at home. It is well-known to them that their flare-ups are caused by a combination of physical, dietary, and environmental factors. Because there is no cure for interstitial cystitis, restricting certain foods and beverages, such as sodas, caffeinated beverages, and citrus fruits and beverages, has been shown to improve symptoms. Apple cider vinegar may help settle the problem in several ways, including:

- providing nutrients that assist the bladder in processing urine;
- minimizing toxicity inside the urine; and
- detoxifying the blood and bodily fluids that are likely involved in the bladder's functioning.

This easy-to-use tonic is a great way to get your daily dose of apple cider vinegar into your system.

- Add 1 tablespoon of apple cider vinegar to 1 cup of water to prepare a drink.

Continue to drink the mixture every hour for as long as the symptoms persist before stopping.

Iron deficiency can be avoided

Iron deficiency is characterized by a deficiency in the number of hemoglobin-rich red blood cells, resulting in oxygen deprivation of organs. Excessive tiredness and sluggishness are common complaints. The body's inability to produce enough red blood cells or excessive bleeding (even strong menstrual flows might constitute excessive bleeding) will also be to blame for the lack of red blood cells. Though iron deficiency anemia symptoms can go unnoticed for a long period of time because of their mildness, many anemia symptoms are strong enough to have a significant impact on a person's day-to-day life.
Symptoms such as fatigue, mood swings, and a weakened immune system occur when the body's ability to absorb

and use iron is impaired. This can have a wide range of effects on the body's various systems.

You can mitigate iron insufficiency by taking an over-the-counter iron supplement. You may help your body absorb iron by taking ACV on a daily basis, which will reduce the need for supplements.

An iron-boosting drink can be made by mixing:

- two cups of water with
- two tablespoons of apple cider vinegar (ACV).
- ½ cup spinach
- ½ cored green apples

Blend all ingredients until well blended in a blender.

Drink every day.

It increases the absorption of calcium

Calcium is an essential element that many people assume they know about, but few are aware of the tremendous effects it has on a number of biological systems. Calcium is well known for its role in bone and tooth development and maintenance. In fact, the bones and teeth contain 99 percent of the body's calcium. That vital mineral, however, could be useful for:

- cognition;
- proper nervous system functioning
- maintaining muscular tissue
- preventing blood circulation;
- pressure difficulties.

Calcium has unquestionably risen to prominence as a critical component in the quest to preserve good health and well-being. You may think you're getting enough calcium in your diet because there are so many calcium-enriched goods on the market, but this isn't always the case. While calcium pills may be beneficial, the best way to get calcium is through a diet rich in calcium-rich foods like apple cider vinegar.

Apple cider vinegar is a far more natural way to ensure that you're getting the maximum amount of calcium from your meals, and it does so by providing two essentials: acetic acid and magnesium, both of which are necessary for maximum absorption of calcium from the foods you eat every day. Acetic acid in ACV helps the body absorb calcium by aiding the breakdown of calcium-rich meals and facilitating digestion. Oxalates, which are found in meals high in calcium, such as dark green vegetables, act as a true block to calcium absorption.

Oxalates are neutralized and calcium absorption is improved by ACV's acetic acid. ACV contains magnesium, which aids in the absorption of calcium.

- 1 cup of calcium-fortified orange juice
- 1 cup distilled water
- 1 tablespoon of apple cider vinegar (ACV).

Drink every day.

Vitamin C deficiencies should be avoided

When you're healthy and well, the systems in your body can operate to their greatest potential. When one's immune system is weak, it's common for people to get sick. Having a compromised immune system leaves you open to a host of other health problems, such as the typical cold, vitamin and mineral deficiencies, and even more serious illnesses. This can happen when antibiotics are used to treat an illness but instead increase parasite growth, causing yeast infections. This can happen when over-the-counter and prescription drugs weaken the immune system's ability to fight off changes in mineral, fluid, and bacterial balances. Definitely, when your body's systems are working together, your immune system is able to perform at a higher level! In light of the fact that apple cider vinegar contains numerous vitamins, minerals, and enzymes that are vital to human health, you should be aware of this. Along with antiviral and antibacterial properties, it assists the body's ability to fight illness while also ensuring optimal physiological function. An important part of reaching this state of peak performance is improving your body's ability to get and use the nutrients it needs.

Adding apple cider vinegar to your diet may help you better absorb vitamin C. By drinking ACV, you may be able to kick-start a beneficial cycle that enhances the body's immunity, increases nutrient absorption, and so on. To make a daily vitamin C-boosting drink, mix the following ingredients:

- Organic apple juice, a single serving
- 1 frozen banana
- frozen strawberries, 1 cup
- ACV and cinnamon, each 1 teaspoon each.

Blend all ingredients together in a food processor or blender until smooth. Once a day, take pleasure in it.

Take Care of Your Vitamin B Deficiency

Vitamin-B is able to ensure the proper operation of a surprising number of different systems. Deficiencies in vitamin B have been linked to depression. Vitamin B helps the body make the right proteins, nourish nerve cells, and provide the elements needed for DNA synthesis, among many other important functions.

Many people don't know how to incorporate more B vitamin-rich foods into their diets to avoid a B vitamin deficit, which is surprising. Spirulina and other B-vitamin-rich foods like chia seeds and avocados are wonderful supplements to any diet that is lacking in these green leafy vegetables. The following ACV tonic may also assist you in maintaining consistent vitamin B levels. Almost any health food store or local food market will have spirulina powder for sale as a dietary supplement.

To mix a cocktail, combine the following ingredients in the following order:

- 1 tablespoon apple cider vinegar
- a cup of distilled water
- 1 pear, cored, and
- 1 teaspoon of spirulina

Using a blender, combine all of the ingredients and blend until you get the desired consistency. Drink every day.

Vitamin B plays other roles in assisting your body:

- It is a mixture of information from carbohydrates and DNA creation that gives you energy. A deficiency can result in neurological difficulties, discomfort, and sensory issues.
- Electrolyte transport requires the development of strength, which riboflavin helps to do by supporting the conversion of fatty acid molecules into energy. Cracked lips, sun sensitivity, and a scratchy throat are symptoms of ariboflavinosis, which can progress to more serious health problems if the vitamin is deficient.
- Niacin facilitates energy-transfer processes in the metabolism of glucose, fat, and alcohol. It can cause anger, sleeplessness, weakness, and dermatitis.

- Fatty acid and carbohydrate oxidation, protein synthesis and biosynthesis, cholesterol and hormone synthesis are all catalyzed by vitamin B (pantothenic acid). Acne is one of the most common signs of insufficiency.
- involved in the synthesis of neurotransmitters and hemoglobin, as well as in the metabolism of proteins and lipids. Anemia, depression, dermatitis, hypertension, and water retention are all symptoms of a deficiency in vitamin B-12.
- Proteins, carbs, and fats are all involved in the metabolism of biotin; it also metabolizes energy, proteins, and cholesterol. Insufficiency causes stunted development and neurological problems in children.
- assists normal cell division, especially during pregnancy, and is critical in the creation of hemoglobin and other blood components. High homocysteine levels can be caused by deficiency, which may lead to delivery issues.
- All cobalamins (different types): Red blood cells are produced in bone marrow, nerve sheaths, and proteins are incorporated into cell metabolism.

Memory loss and other cognitive issues are the final results of anemia.

Irritable Bowel Syndrome (IBS)

Chronic constipation, which can be a symptom of Irritable Bowel Syndrome (IBS), can cause a person to experience discomfort when digesting meals. Diarrhea, constipation, or both are common symptoms for people with IBS, in addition to the pain that they feel during digestion. IBS treatments, which range from natural to pharmaceutical and number in the hundreds, do not have a known cause. There are hundreds of them.

IBS medications, like many pharmaceutical treatments, have certain undesired side effects that have led many people with the condition to seek out more natural options. Apple cider vinegar's use as an all-natural IBS pain reliever continues to grow due to its antiviral and antibacterial properties, as well as its specific acids that neutralize digestive enzymes and gastric acid. Pectin, a dietary fiber, also helps soften and bulk up stools for easier passage from the colon. In addition to being an inexpensive and accessible therapy, apple cider vinegar

(ACV) is packed with immune-boosting vitamins, minerals, enzymes, and natural phytochemicals.

Combining the following ingredients will yield a preventive tonic:

- 1 tablespoon of ACV
- 2 cups of water

Prevent IBS by drinking this combination before meals.

Combine the following ingredients for an effective tonic that alleviates existing symptoms:

- 2-4 teaspoons of ACV
- A cup of water

Sip slowly over the course of thirty minutes.

It improves the diets of vegetarians

There is a significant risk associated with a vegetarian diet that some vital nutrients may not be able to pass through. Vegetarians can be broken down into a few different groups based on the foods they don't eat:

• A "vegetarian" (one who does not eat meat but consumes dairy products, eggs, and animal products)

- A “vegan” (who does not eat all products created from animals).

Vegetarians and vegans are two different things.

If you don't eat meat or animal products, you can get the micronutrients your body needs from a vegetarian or vegan diet.

Vegetarians and vegans may be able to follow a well-thought-out diet to meet their food needs.

The benefits of incorporating apple cider vinegar into a vegan or vegetarian diet include:

- Nutritional absorption of macronutrients (such as carbs) as well as micronutrients in the diet is made possible through this.
- The fiber in ACV aids digestion, making it easier to digest plant-based meals, which is common in vegetarian diets.This helps to ensure appropriate cell functioning and growth. ACV contains phytonutrients and enzymes that have antiviral and antibacterial capabilities, enhancing the disease-fighting abilities of a plant-based diet that is vegetarian (which might be without immunity-

boosting vitamins typically found in dairy food and healthy meat).

A blender is all you need to produce a calcium-boosting drink:

- ½ tablespoon of ACV
- 1 cup of coconut or almond milk
- Your favorite fruits and spices

Drink every day.

Chapter 4

Apple Cider Vinegar Uses for Healthy Hair

Do you regularly invest a lot of time and money into your hair care routine?

No matter how much effort you put into maintaining your hair, you may wind up with unkempt locks that don't meet your expectations.

Do you think it's becoming more difficult to keep your hair's natural beauty intact?

Want to stop spending money on chemical-laden hair products that claim to be good for the environment but fail miserably?

When you think about how many hair products you use on a regular basis for shampooing and styling, you can only imagine how much residue is left behind.

When a product is designed to help hair grow, shine, body, highlights, and more, the residue it leaves behind actually impedes natural growth, shine, and more! Your hair's follicles, cuticles, pores, and ends may be damaged to the point that no product can save them from becoming unmanageable and unhealthy.

You've found it: apple cider vinegar will bring your hair back to health and give you the hair you've always wanted! ACV is a great source of naturally occurring acids, enzymes, vitamins, and nutrients that work together to support healthy hair. To get more brilliant and longer-lasting color treatments that are safe to drink, these ingredients may be found in various formulations with functional capabilities that range from a clarifying rinse or shampoo.

You may simply get the results you desire with these easy-to-create and simple-to-use treatments supported by scientific explanations of how and why this product, together with the combinations and treatments for each individual benefit, helps to eradicate the hair concerns you struggle with on a daily basis.

The conclusion is that if you want to get the results you've been hoping for for a long time, are fed up with spending money on products and treatments that don't work, and want to utilize an all-natural solution, apple cider vinegar is the way to go. Implementing these ACV treatments now can help you restore damaged hair and get you closer to having the gorgeous hair you've always wanted.

Help with Hair Loss

Having thinning hair can be embarrassing, and it's not simply a problem for the elderly. Increasing numbers of women of all ages are searching for ways to halt the thinning of their hair. Prescription and over-the-counter medications often contain dangerous chemicals and additives that can cause health problems and exacerbate existing medical conditions.

To get the benefits of baldness treatments safely and successfully, look no further than a bottle of apple cider vinegar. You can:

- Improve the blood circulation in your scalp by employing apple cider vinegar as a fantastic remedy for thinning hair.
- Improve the flow of blood to the roots of hair.
- Ensure that critical nutrients are delivered to the scalp in an efficient manner.

ACV's health-enhancing properties aid in promoting hair regrowth and halting the progression of baldness. As well as having important elements for healthy hair, ACV also gives your skin the nutrition it needs to keep your hair shaft in good shape.

To make a hair tonic, mix together:

- 2 tablespoons ACV.
- 1 tablespoon of drinking water.
- 1/2 teaspoon cayenne pepper.

Five minutes of rubbing the mixture into the scalp is all that's required to properly apply this to thinning hair. Before shampooing, leave it on the scalp for one hour. Within two to four weeks, you should see some progress.

It's possible that cayenne's two chemical constituents, capsaicin and quercetin, are responsible for promoting hair growth by stimulating the roots of hair and increasing blood flow to the scalp.

Creating a hair shampoo

Some hair-care products actually deliver on their promises, while others leave behind unsightly residue and buildup around the roots of hair, hair shafts, and the scalp. There is a risk that this buildup will cause excessive oiliness, uncontrollable frizz, or a disappointing color. As if that wasn't bad enough, many products for your hair say they can get rid of this buildup by using harsh chemicals and abrasives. In reality, they dry your hair and make it even more difficult to manage.

By using apple cider vinegar as a rinse during your routine washing and conditioning treatments, you may easily eliminate residue and restore your hair's health, shine, and color naturally and without undesired adverse effects by using apple cider vinegar as a rinse. Using apple cider vinegar to remove buildup and debris from the hair does

not harm the follicles or upset the scalp's pH balance because of its cleansing acids and enzymes.
Make a hair rinse by mixing 1 cup of water with half a cup of apple cider vinegar.

Apply it to the hair when you shampoo and condition it, as you normally would. Rinse with warm water after allowing the mixture to sit on the hair and scalp for five minutes. In order to keep hair from becoming weighed down by buildup, repeat this method with each subsequent wash.

Shampoo Manufacturing

Some shampoos leave your hair feeling weighed down, dry, or loaded with frizz, while others leave your hair bouncy, shiny, and free of frizz. It can be costly, time-consuming, and harmful to your hair to compare several brands. You may use apple cider vinegar as a shampoo alternative to clean your hair organically and return it to its lustrous and healthy state. You may see a significant improvement in the quality of your hair with just one treatment!

ACV is a low-cost, natural alternative that is free of toxic chemicals and other additives that could increase the frequency flowing hair with these excellent benefits:

- Cleanse your hair of buildup and filth with the help of apple cider vinegar.
- Increase the volume, bounce, and shine of your hair and scalp by massaging in nutrients and vitamins.
- Provide pH-neutralizing enzymes as well as therapeutic proteins.
- aims to increase access to hair health insurance and enhance the appearance of individual hairs.
- Use a scrubbing motion to gently remove environmental residues.

In order to create shampoo, add these to a bottle:

- 1/2 cup ACV + 2 tablespoon lemon juice
- A cup of water

Instead of shampoo, use the mixture to massage the mixture into the scalp and strands before washing and going on to condition.

A substitute for your usual shampoo should be used every time you wash your hair, or you can use it in conjunction with your regular shampoo.

Get to Work on Your Air Conditioner

Deep conditioning treatments, as well as balms and solutions that claim to leave hair silky and hydrated, are now available both at home and in salons. It's hard to keep up with all the conditioning treatments. Certain types of conditioners may not deliver on their promises, whether the hair is generally greasy, dry, curly, or straight.

As it turns out, the same bottle of apple cider vinegar you use for your normal tonics also does wonders for your feminine health and vitality! If used as a conditioner, it could benefit hair of all hues, textures, and types. In spite of the fact that many treatment choices are available, few supply you with the nutrients included in ACV, and hence are as inexpensive as ACV and produce results following an initial treatment as ACV does. Together with the additional conditioning of coconut oil, ACV is a powerful conditioner that combats frizziness, battles knots, and keeps hair shiny while adjusting the pH of the scalp.

Add all the ingredients to a bottle and shake to combine.

- ½ cup of ACV
- ½ cup essential coconut oil
- 1 cup of water

Afterwards, cover your hair with a shower cap and wait 30 minutes for the mask to work. After that, wash and dry your hair to reveal a new head of hair that is full of vitality.

Preventing Baldness

Hereditary factors, frequent hair damage treatments, and a lack of nutrition that promotes healthy hair growth are all possible causes of baldness.

If left unfiltered, ACV's naturally occurring enzymes, proteins, vitamins, minerals, and acids combine to:

- Add cleansing and restorative materials to the foundation of baldness;
- Remove aggravating reasons that may contribute to hair loss. Hair and scalp problems can be improved by fostering new growth and maintaining the health of this growth.

Cosmetics that contain chemicals in the hair-regeneration process can irritate the scalp and cause damage while also interfering with the body's ability to absorb and use critical nutrients for healthy hair re-growth. All shampoos, conditioners, and treatments like apple cider vinegar (ACV) should only be made with natural ingredients.

If you want to get rid of baldness and keep your body healthy, you need to apply both a topical ACV treatment and an ACV tonic.

A tonic can be made by combining:

- ½ cup of water;
- ½ cup of apple cider vinegar
- ½ tsp. cayenne powder.

Dot balding patches with this concoction by rubbing it in from the roots up to the scalp. When finished, rinse with shampoo and follow with conditioner as you normally would. Three: the procedure shows results in as little as two to four weeks when repeated frequently.

Add one tablespoon of apple cider vinegar (ACV) to a cup of water to make a drinkable tonic.

Drink on a daily basis.

Vitamins, minerals, enzymes, and acids found in apple cider vinegar (ACV) are included in this solution, which:

- Supports the fitness of systems directly related to hair development and health, such as metabolism and blood circulation.
- Some B vitamins, vitamin C, vitamin D, and iron may contribute to baldness if a deficiency is not addressed.

Hair Straightening

After a shower, if your hair is a tangled mess and you can't simply brush or comb it, you might consider using a detangling solution. Because of their claims to leave hair shiny and free of knots, many treatments on the market contain chemicals or unnatural ingredients that can actually strip the hair of its natural oils and leave it looking dull and damaged. ACV is an effective tangle-buster that doesn't harm hair health. Besides restoring vital vitamins and minerals, ACV helps decrease knots by removing residue from cleaning chemicals while hydrating and conditioning your hair strands and making styling easier.

Dissolve the following in a spray bottle for detangling spray:

- 1/2 cup of ACV.
- A cup of water

Comb and detangle hair after spraying it with this solution on your scalp and brushing it thoroughly.

Reduce Stiffness

Frizzy hair is a frustrating condition that can be caused by environmental factors such as humidity or wind, or by prolonged exposure to potentially harmful ingredients in hair care and styling products. Because the strands of hair remain open, they are unable to absorb moisture, and this is the root cause of frizzy hair. Hair that has been blow-dried makes it more susceptible to the effects of the weather and styling products and treatments that cause it to look "frizzy."

Spot-treating frizziness and enjoying healthy, lustrous, manageable hair are both made possible by the incorporation of naturally therapeutic proteins and nutrients into your hair strands. Many "natural" products on the market have preservatives or synthetic elements that can cause hair damage, even if they are branded *"natural."* Apple cider vinegar is an excellent solution for frizzy hair that saves you from having to deal with it all the time. ACV is full of proteins and enzymes, which can help your hair stay healthy.

Combine the following ingredients in a bottle for an anti-frizz treatment in the shower:

- ½ cup of ACV
- ½ cup of water
- 2 teaspoons of liquid coconut oil.

Apply the mixture to your hair and let it sit for five minutes after you've finished conditioning it in the shower. After rinsing off the solution, dry your hair as you normally would.

In a spray container, combine the following ingredients to create a prestyling, frizz-fighting solution:

- 1 cup of water
- ½ cup of apple cider vinegar.

Using the ACV spray, saturate damp hair. Towel-dry and

style as usual after allowing the spray to sit for five minutes.

Prevent Split Ends

Split ends occur when the hair's finish splits into two strands, causing the hair to split from the bottom up when tested. Both the appearance and hair care and styling can be made more difficult or frustrating as a result of this damage to the hair. Split ends can be avoided and healthy hair protected from split-end damage if you just clip the ends of your hair once a month. Another strategy for minimizing breakage is to maintain an adequate intake of nutrients that promote healthy hair growth, like silica, calcium, vitamin C, and vitamins B and B complex.

Getting enough vitamins and minerals will make your hair healthier from the inside out and help you avoid getting split ends. Using all-natural, unfiltered, organic apple cider vinegar as an ingested preventative step and a localized therapy for split ends is the most efficient way to deal with split ends.

In order to get the most out of your vitamins and minerals, Combine:

- 1 cup of water
- 1 tablespoon of ACV

Drink every day.

Split ends can be treated with a mixture of:

- ½ cup water
- ½ cup ACV
- ¼ cup mashed avocado

Rinse well after 30 minutes and reapply to the bottom 1/4 of your hair. Split ends can be prevented in as little as a few weeks if you do this treatment several times a week.

Get rid and prevent Headlice

Having to deal with head lice may be a tedious and difficult experience, especially when it affects a large percentage of the population that is of school age. Head lice are easily spread among large groups of people, such as a classroom full of youngsters. Head lice can be efficiently prevented by limiting one's contact with people who have been verified to be infected with the parasite. A confirmed head lice infestation necessitates not only immediate treatment but also preventative steps to guarantee that any remaining lice are killed before they can re-infest your home. Several over-the-counter medications are available to treat head lice. However, the majority of them contain synthetic and chemical ingredients that may be harmful to your overall health or dangerous to adults and children with certain skin sensitivities. Try ACV as an all-natural option.

Lice treatment in advance:

Put a shower cap on your hair and apply undiluted apple cider vinegar to the scalp and hair. Wait at least 4-5 hours before shampooing. After removing the cap and thoroughly rinsing the hair with water, use a fine-tooth comb to remove the nits and eggs from the hair.

Continue doing this every day until the lice and eggs have all died.

Maintain and boost hair growth

The number of hair-growth products on the market is enormous, and it's likely to grow even larger in the coming years. Chemical components, "all-natural" promises, or guarantees that growth will follow the product's use can all distinguish one product from another. The particular results may vary from product to product and individual to individual, depending on a number of factors. You can boost your hair regrowth naturally by using ACV in combination with a variety of other hair-growth methods. Due to its high quantities of important minerals and vitamins, apple cider vinegar is touted for a wide range of health benefits. Every drop of ACV contains natural acids, enzymes, and proteins, making it a highly efficient treatment for hair loss and support for hair regrowth. You can keep your hair healthy by massaging your scalp regularly, eating a diet rich in protein, and limiting your hair's exposure to heat treatments and hazardous chemical compounds.

The following ingredients can be mixed together to create a hair growth treatment that can be used on a nightly basis:

- ½ cup of apple cider vinegar
- 1-2 cups of aloe vera juice.

Apply the mixture to the scalp and all the way down to the ends of the hair, then cover with a shower cap and let it sit on the hair for 7-8 hours. Take a daily shower or hair rinse. In as little as 2-4 weeks, you can improve the health of your hair, restore important nutrients naturally, and learn to obtain the results of your efforts.

Get Rid of Water Hardness Debris

If you're talking about water that contains minerals from rocks and sediments in your community, the process of getting water, or between treatment and your home, you can use the term "hard water." Hard water is to blame if your hair is discolored, smelly, or difficult to maintain, even after you shampoo.

A remedy pump or filter that removes the minerals from the water is the simplest technique to improve hard water. However, these may be prohibitively expensive and ineffectual. Even if you want to treat your water in the long run, treating flowing hair is essential if you want to get rid of the hard water effects as quickly as possible. Choosing an all-natural treatment like ACV instead of a chemical-laden over-the-counter treatment for hard water hair may be your safest and most successful option. Apple cider vinegar is one of the safest and most effective ways to remove buildup and residue from hair. ACV is just as powerful as top-of-the-line solutions at removing mineral buildup, but it can do so quickly, safely, and without endangering the health of your hair or skin.

Acidic apple cider vinegar, which is rich in nutrients, can help restore important minerals and vitamins to your hair's cuticles and shafts, as well as reverse the damage caused by calcium deposits. What's the most exciting part?
To remove buildup from hair, the enzymes and acids in ACV can be used.

Use the following ingredients to prepare an ACV hair rinse:

- a single cup of water
- 1 cup of ACV

After shampooing and conditioning your hair as usual, follow up with an excellent hair treatment. Rinse your hair after 5 minutes of the solution remaining on your hair.

The recipes in this book for homemade shampoo and conditioner can help you make your own if you don't want to use products that are full of chemicals.

Add some radiance

The dullness of one's hair is one of the most common complaints, and the hair care industry is well aware of this. Numerous products, ranging in price from $1 to over $100, are available to help dull hair regain its light-reflective sheen. These things can be bought at your favorite supermarket, drugstore, salon, or hair product supplier.

If you want to revive dull hair and give it the lustrous sheen we associate with healthy hair, all you need is an apple cider vinegar bottle.

Your hair's condition and appearance can be improved by incorporating apple cider vinegar into your daily diet and hair care regimen. You can:

- Restore the natural balance of nutrients in your body's systems that promote hair health by removing styling product residue and build-up.
- Restore damaged hair caused by heat and chemical damage through styling, coloring, or treatments.

For lustrous hair, add to a cup of water 1 teaspoon apple cider vinegar

Drinking on a regular basis can help you keep your hair in good condition by providing the necessary nutrients.

Make a topical hair solution by mixing:

- 1 cup of normal water
- 1 cup of ACV
- A teaspoon of peppermint extract

Apply the ideal solution to your hair and straighten strands after shampooing and conditioning. Rinse well after allowing the mixture to sit for 5-10 minutes.

In addition to helping to repair damage and restore a healthy sheen, this procedure can help restore hair health at the cellular level, as well as at the pore and cuticle levels.

Hair Colors

For the same attractive results as chemical treatments, you can use ACV in place of the more expensive and hair-damaging ones if you're looking for natural at-home solutions to highlight flowing hair. When exposed to sunshine, the acids and enzymes in ACV help lighten hair naturally. In order to get the results you want, you only need to use ACV in combination with other activities that make your skin light and smooth.

Combining the following ingredients, both at room temperature, will produce an effective hair lightener:

- 1 cup of drinking water
- ½ cup of fresh-squeezed lemon juice
- ½ cup of liquid coconut oil
- ½ cup of ACV

Apply it to the hair and allow it to sit in the sun for 20 to 30 minutes. Natural, affordable, and effective results can be achieved under one treatment using this procedure.

Chlorine Damage Can Be Reversed

Swimming in a chlorinated pool during the summer months can cause hair to turn dark green, dry out, and become brittle and brittle, turning even the most gorgeous tresses into a mess of unmanageable frizz and split ends. What is the protective remedy used if you can't stand the pool and can't take the considered chlorine damage? What kind of treatment can both undo and avoid the harm caused by chlorine?

What is a low-cost, no-visit salon treatment that may be used every day without damaging hair? Vinegar is made from the juice of apples.

Natural elements in apple cider vinegar close the hair shaft appropriately, preventing the strands from chemical harm like chlorine damage, creating the ideal environment for hair to block entering pollutants that might degrade hair quality from the inside out. Additionally, apple cider vinegar is a natural cleaner that can eliminate dirt and chemical buildup from hair while also removing the green chlorine shine from even the lightest of blondes.

In a spray bottle, combine the following ingredients to create a chlorine-busting rinse:

The recipe calls for

1 cup of plain water and 2 cups of apple cider vinegar.

When you shampoo and rinse your hair, apply the mixture to your hair before and after exposing it to chlorine.

Healthy Scalp Promotion

Alternatives to synthetic products that promise to make your hair and scalp healthier include apple cider vinegar

(ACV). No matter how slight or severe your scalp health condition is, this is a quick, low-cost solution that is packed with nutrients. Your mood is directly influenced by the health of your scalp. Scalp health is a serious business, and you'll find this out by talking to someone who has severe dandruff, bouts of hair loss, or an itchy scalp on a regular basis. It's easy to see that scalp health is a lucrative business, with a wide variety of products on the market that promise to restore health to the scalp at a price. Many scalp-restorative products don't meet your expectations or cost more than you thought they would. This is because the products are hard to use or because your health problems are made worse by the chemicals or synthetic ingredients in them.

Combine the following for a healthy scalp:

- One cup of water
- half a cup of apple cider vinegar
- 1 teaspoon cayenne pepper
- 1 teaspoon organic honey

Apply the mixture to wet hair and massage it into the scalp until it is well absorbed. 30 minutes before rinsing, shampooing, and conditioning, apply the mixture to hair and scalp. Repeat on a weekly or daily basis.

Remove Product Residue

Besides shampoo, conditioner, straightening and curling products, keratin and emollients such as gels and sprays, mousses and leave-in conditioners, do you use any other hair care products to color or style your hair? The large majority of people who replied yes are likely to have a significant amount of product residue on their hair. Despite the fact that you may not be able to detect a chemical residue after washing your hair, styling products and treatments used to clean, condition, or cure beautiful hair may leave behind a film that you cannot see just by looking at or touching it.

There are hundreds of people who use clarifying treatments that claim to remove the unhealthy buildup from flowing hair, but you may be surprised to hear that most of them only partially fix the problem and that several can leave behind more residue. Rather than using harsh chemicals or additives that may take nutrients and buildup, consider using ACV to cleanse your hair with conviction. Apple cider vinegar's naturally occurring clarifying enzymes and acids make it an effective, yet safe, treatment for removing blemishes. It is possible to remove residue left behind by hair products and follow up with an application rich in therapeutic nutrients that may leave your hair healthier than before with this suggested treatment of two different applications of ACV for your hair.

The following ingredients should be combined to make an ACV soak:

- 1 cup of ACV
- 1/2 cup of water

Using a shower cap, cover your hair with an appropriate solution and let the combination sit on your hair for 30 minutes. You can have a normal shower after rinsing with drinking water, but don't add any product to your hair.

Mix ½ cup apple cider vinegar with ½ cup of liquid coconut oil and ½ cup of water to make a nourishing conditioner.

Apply this mixture to your hair and scalp and massage it in for two hours after rinsing out the ACV soak. Leave it on for 30 minutes, then rinse it out with a normal amount of water. Towel dry and comb.

Chapter 5

Apple Cider Vinegar for Skincare

Skincare is a multibillion-dollar industry, and millions of women all over the world contribute to it. Our skin is bombarded with reminders of our wrinkles, blemishes, redness, liver spots, and varicose veins questionnaire, along with messages that people can be proactive in reversing the effects of aging and improving their beauty by paying a few dollars here and a few dollars there for products designed to help us declare victory in the war of skin conditions that will make it less attractive. Before you spend another penny on the newest and best skin-care product, read this amazing thing about apple cider vinegar.

Organic apple cider vinegar can be used to improve and restore the fitness of skin, and this chapter focuses on a number of applications you can simply and quickly execute to renew your skin layer and feel better about yourself. In the comfort of your own home, apple cider vinegar can help you attain long-lasting beauty without the need for chemicals, additives, or synthetic products that could cause more harm than good.

The best part about apple cider vinegar is the nourishment it can provide your skin. Acai berry juice (ACV) contains potent antioxidant vitamins that help repair skin damage and help prevent additional damage due to unfavorable changes in skin cells. In addition to improving your skin's health and appearance, apple cider vinegar has minerals that boost blood flow and circulation, making it a better option. This natural ingredient's ability to keep the skin clear and clean without causing significant adverse effects is only another perk.

It reduces the symptoms of psoriasis

Psoriasis is a painful and ugly skin disorder that is thought to be caused by trauma to the skin layer, stress, smoking, excessive alcohol intake, sun exposure, and some medications. Non-contagious, psoriasis is characterized by a silver or red patch of skin that may or may not itch.

The autoimmune system views your skin layer cells as pathogens and overstimulates the creation of skin cells as a response. Even though many lotions sold over the counter can help with your psoriasis or treat your skin condition, many contain harsh ingredients or have unpleasant side effects that could make your skin even more sensitive to the lotion. This could make your condition even worse.

Any psoriasis treatment can benefit from lifestyle changes that reduce the elements that are thought to contribute to the condition (such as stopping smoking and limiting alcohol use, sun exposure, and stress). Psoriasis sufferers have taken to using apple cider vinegar as a treatment because of the many beneficial ingredients it provides, both internally and at the site of irritation. ACV contains vitamin C, which boosts immunity; enzymes, which improve blood quality; and antioxidants that repair damage.

As a result, all-natural apple cider vinegar can help your skin stay healthy and keep your body's skin-supporting systems in good shape as a result.

To produce a topical therapy, combine:

- ½ cup of water
- ½ cup of ACV.

For 30 minutes, place a cloth soaked in the solution on the affected area.

Combine 1 cup of water with 1 tablespoon of apple cider vinegar to make a drink that promotes healthy skin.

Drink every day.

Hemorrhoids are alleviated.

Although they are more common in the elderly and pregnant women, people of all ages are susceptible to hemorrhoids. Haemorrhoids, which are inflamed veins that can be internal or external and can be exceedingly uncomfortable or merely irritating, are most often caused by straining or pressing the bowels during defecating. In mild situations, hemorrhoids are not a cause for concern, but in more serious ones, surgery may be necessary. They can be treated in many different ways, from applying lotion to swallowing digestive aids, all of which can help with the symptoms but also address the underlying cause. Try apple cider vinegar as a natural alternative to chemical-laden OTC remedies that may cause constipation or diarrhea or worsen the condition. Hemorrhoids may benefit from apple cider vinegar's restorative properties, which are said to be superior to those of over-the-counter remedies. Digestive aids in ACV like pectin and acetic and malic acids work together to bind waste and lubricate the stools, lowering the strain on the colon during defecation and decreasing the risk of hemorrhoids by facilitating waste movement through the digestive tract better.

To make a hemorrhoid-healing drink, mix 1 cup of water with 1 tablespoon of apple cider vinegar.

Drink three times a day. Within 30 minutes, you'll feel the benefits of this potent combo.

For topical relief, Combine:

- 1/2 cup of water
- 1/2 cup of ACV.

Apply the mixture to the affected region as needed with a cotton ball or soft cloth soaked in the mixture to reduce inflammation and relieve pain.

Cleanses Your Pores

See how many pollutants your face is subjected to on a single day. The appearance and health of your skin are harmed by exposure to pollutants in the air and to visible dirt and grime. Touching someone's face with your hands—consciously or subconsciously—is a major component in the formation of clogged pores; this is something you probably do many times each day. Your skin may become oily, greasy, or overly dry if your pores become clogged with harmful deposits from your own hands.

Many commercially available cleansers contain harsh or abrasive ingredients that can disrupt the skin's normal oil and pH balance, resulting in unhygienic or unpleasant skin disorders. Apple cider vinegar, a natural alternative to chemical-laden treatments, has cleansing capabilities that remove unwanted deposits from the face while also keeping the skin's pores open and healthy. By restoring the natural pH balance of your skin, ACV has also been proven to regulate the oils made by the skin, producing a healthier balance of oil production and minimizing the clogging of pores.

To produce a pore cleaner, combine these within a bowl:

- ½ cup of warm water
- ½ cup of ACV

Use a facecloth to soak up the liquid, wring out the excess, then gently wipe your skin with the towel to get rid of any remaining residue. Rinse and reabsorb the ACV mixture many times, and then reapply it to your skin until it seems clear and revitalized.

Improve your skin tone

Instead of shelling out big bucks for expensive skin toners, try apple cider vinegar instead! ACV is a fantastic solution for treating skin concerns because it has the same active ingredients that make it beneficial for addressing health and wellness issues. In most cases, the goal of using a toner is to remove dead skin cells and oil from the face to reveal a clean, clear, and supple layer of skin.

Because of the vitamins and naturally occurring acids in ACV, it is a powerful and safe way to improve the appearance of skin while also restoring the skin's pH and oil balance. Acne and unsightly blemishes can be treated with apple cider vinegar's acetic and malic acids, which provide antioxidant benefits and help restore the health of skin cells and reverse oxidative damage. Apple cider vinegar also helps balance the pH levels of your skin, remove dirt and oils from your pores, and treat acne.

Skin toner:

- ½ cup of lukewarm water
- ½ cup of ACV

Apply a cotton ball soaked in the ideal solution to your facial and neck skin. All of the other mixes can be stored in an airtight container at night in a cool, dark place.

Reduce the Intensity of Jellyfish Stings

Jellyfish stings are a little-known fact, and it's unclear why they may be so painful. The tentacles of jellyfish are used to discharge nematocysts, which cling to your skin and then release toxins into your blood. It is possible to have minor to agonizing discomfort as a result of nematocysts, as well as the need for medical assistance if breathing or vision are impaired. The most common treatment for jellyfish stings that aren't as bad but are still unpleasant is to apply urine to the area that was stung.

Although certain jellyfish stings can be alleviated with the use of urine, ACV is an all-natural substitute that might relax your skin layer by releasing the tentacles and supplying the required nutrients to your skin layer for immediate repair. Apple cider vinegar contains acetic acid, which can be used in two ways to alleviate the pain of jellyfish stings:

1. When there is less inflammation, the tentacles can come out of the skin, and toxic substances can't get into the bloodstream.
2. Using the sting immediately and efficiently to neutralize the reaction within your skin, bloodstream, and nerves, relieving pain.

Apply undiluted ACV to the sting site to create a topical solution.

You can reapply as many times as necessary.

While you're still in pain, combine the following to make a glass or two:

- 1 tablespoon of ACV
- 1 cup of water

Take a sip every hour for the next four hours to help reduce inflammation, give your skin the vitamins and minerals it needs to repair itself, and help your body get rid of toxins.

Ease Sunburn

Overexposure to the sun's rays can cause inflammation that is not only uncomfortable and ugly, but also potentially harmful to your skin. There is a growing body of evidence linking excessive exposure to the sun to skin cancers and other abnormal growths. The fastest and easiest way to soothe and repair sunburned skin is to use natural ingredients that help cells grow and repair.

Several skin-health products on the market claim to contain vitamin C, which is one of the most efficient agents for enhancing cellular health. Few of the cosmetic solutions on the market support the combination of components provided by apple cider vinegar that may promote skin health organically, safely, and efficiently. After sunburn, ACV helps soothe the tightening and burning by restoring the skin's natural acid-enzyme balance through its beneficial acids and enzymes. Topical use of ACV boosts your skin's vitamin C levels and protects it from free radical damage that could lead to malignant cell changes, which is why you should use it.

Combine the following ingredients to create a skin soak:

- ½ cup of cool water
- ½ cup of ACV

Using a wet towel or sponge, apply the ACV mixture to the skin around the item.

Soak for 30 minutes in a tub filled with water and 2 cups of apple cider vinegar.

To make a drink, combine the following ingredients in the following order:

- 1 cup of water or orange juice straight from the squeezer
- Organic aloe vera juice, one tablespoonful at a time.
- 1 tablespoon of ACV

Every day, take the mixture three times.

Using these three treatments together can help relieve sunburn symptoms and treat cell damage caused by the sun.

Nail fungus control

In addition to bacteria, viruses, and germs, did you know that apple cider vinegar is an effective fungicide?

ACV has unique applications and benefits that far outweigh those of prescription and over-the-counter medicines. It can be taken orally or used on the outside to treat and prevent fungal nail infections.

ACV is a natural source that delivers:

- Antifungal agents and also a collection of immunity-boosting vitamins.

- Minerals that help you using the reparation and healthy growth of nails.
- Antioxidants that help prevent further and future fungal growth.

To make a drink, add:

1 cup of water and 1 tablespoon of apple cider vinegar to a cup and stir well.

Drinking regularly can be used to treat and prevent disease.

As a fungicide, ACV has been shown to be effective when administered directly to the fungus's source. The ACV soaks into the nail's pores and treats the surrounding nail as it seeps under the nail.

Pour undiluted ACV into a small basin to produce a nail soak.

Allow the nails to rest for 15–30 minutes at the same time for another hour before the fungus diminishes.

Eczema can be reduced

Eczema is a long-term skin condition that causes red, itchy patches of skin. Doctors have categorized eczema as an immunological condition because of the irritation caused by allergens. Since there is no known cure for eczema, there are a plethora of therapies available to help reduce the frequency with which the condition appears and the associated symptoms. It may be that your eczema is caused by an allergy, and cutting back on your exposure to it will help ease the symptoms.

Apple cider vinegar is an all-natural alternative to the many over-the-counter eczema relief solutions on the market. Eczema sufferers can use apple cider vinegar (ACV) to reduce inflammation, keep the eczema-inflamed area clear of irritating external components, and encourage the healing of the skin cells affected by the reaction. ACV also supplies necessary nutrients and hypoallergenic characteristics.

To create a topical therapy, use the following ingredients in equal proportions:

- Water
- ACV

For 30 minutes, immerse a towel in the solution and place it on the affected area.

In order to prepare a drink, you'll need the following ingredients:

- 1 cup of freshly juiced strawberries

- 1 tablespoon of ACV

Drink everyday.

Vitamin C, acetic, and malic acids work together to support a healthy immune system and skin cell repair.

It cleans and pushes away infections from cuts

As a result of a cut or abrasion, infection is the most serious outcome. Irritating substances such as bacteria and viruses can enter the bloodstream and cause infection at the location of the cut as well as throughout the entire body when skin is still exposed. Using hot water and soap to clean the area completely and applying a bandage to the wound are two of the most important and effective ways to prevent infection.

In order to protect both your health and the wound, the following measures should be taken:

1. *There are no foreign poisons in the wound.*
2. *Your defense mechanisms are in full effect.*

Both of these health advantages are possible with apple cider vinegar. It's packed with antiseptic, antiviral, and antibacterial qualities. Assailants with disease-fighting

capabilities may be fought off using apple cider vinegar, and the wound would be protected from future germ exposure. As a way to speed up the healing process, ACV has powerful antioxidants that help regenerate skin cells.
One tablespoon of water and one tablespoon of apple cider vinegar can be used to make a good treatment for your skin.
While cleaning the area, it interacts with the wound to provide further protection against infection and assist the natural healing process.

After cleaning the wound, taking a daily dose of apple cider vinegar (ACV) will help boost your immune system and protect you from bacteria that enter the cut and move through the bloodstream. ACV's powerful vitamins, minerals, and nutrients fight off free radicals and pollutants in the blood, leaving the body healthy and able to heal itself quickly.

Combine 1 cup of water with 1 spoonful of ACV to make the drink.
As the wound continues to heal, drink everyday.

Soothes Diaper Rash

The term "diaper rash" is most commonly used to describe the discomfort felt by a baby's backside as a result of damp or soiled diaper conditions. Diaper rash in adults can be caused by the same reasons that cause diaper rash in babies' bottoms. In adults, "diaper rash" is almost always caused by:

- not cleaning the genitals and anus after using the bathroom; and
- wearing tight-fitting clothes that make it hard for the nether regions to "breathe." This makes it hard for newborns and adults to live their lives in general.

In spite of the fact that many lotions and powders claim to alleviate the problem, ACV not only alleviates symptoms but also helps repair and restore the health of the skin. Because ACV has antiseptic, antibacterial, antifungal, and antiviral properties, it helps keep your skin free of irritating and infection-causing stimuli. This is because it has vitamins, minerals, and antioxidants that help your skin cells grow back.

Make a topical therapy by mixing:

- ½ cup of ACV

- ½ cup of water

Every quarter-hour for two hours, gently touch the affected area with a cotton ball or soft towel that has been soaked in the solution.

Insect Bites Can Be Treated

An insect bite or sting can trigger a variety of reactions, ranging from the slightly annoying to the potentially lethal. While not life-threatening, some insect stings and bites can cause skin disorders such as itchiness, burning, or stinging. These symptoms can continue for days or even weeks. Apple cider vinegar can be used to cure bites and potentially prevent them in the future. Apple cider vinegar's naturally occurring acids and enzymes deter biting and stinging bugs. Bugs are deterred from even approaching someone who has ACV on their skin because they can smell and taste the various elements of ACV from afar.

This is what you'll need to put together a bug spray:

- 1 cup of ACV
- ½ cup of water

You can apply a combination to your skin or use a towel to get the same effect and keep mosquitoes away from stinging or biting you.

Apply undiluted ACV to your skin layer every quarter hour using a towel or cotton ball to form a topical therapy for relieving stings and bites. In addition to preventing swelling at the site of the sting or bite, this can also help neutralize the venom released by the insect that stung or bit you.

If you have any reason to believe that your reaction necessitates medical assistance, seek it without delay.

Reduces Skin's Exposure to the Facial Mask

Apple cider vinegar and other health-restoring items like a nose and mouth mask can help alleviate skin irritation symptoms like redness, acne, or discoloration while also enhancing the overall health of the skin. Because of the acetic and malic acids in apple cider vinegar, your skin's natural oil production (on your face and neck) will be more balanced, and you'll be able to unclog pores and remove dirt from your face from your daily activities. ACV helps your skin's pH balance, which has a big impact on acne sufferers' skin irritation and the number of breakouts and blemishes they get.

Vitamin C and beta carotene are abundant in ACV, making it a potent weapon against free radical damage to the skin at the cellular level. This helps keep your skin healthy and prevents future damage from things like tobacco, UV light, and pollution.

Mash these items into a paste to create a skin-beneficial mask:

- ½ cup of ACV
- ½ of just a single avocado
- 1 tablespoon of natural, unprocessed, organic honey, The honey should be raw and natural.

Rinse off the mask with warm water after 15–30 minutes of application on the skin.

Antioxidants, healthy fats, vitamins, minerals, and enzymes are all found in this blend. All of these can be absorbed by the skin and help the blood flow and:

- heal damage, and restore skin health
- Balance the skin's pH and oil production.
- Cleanse the skin's surface and pores of debris and germs.

Lessen Age Spots

Long-term exposure to sunlight can cause brown or tan oval spots on your skin, which are known as age spots. People over the age of forty are more likely to experience hyperpigmented reactions, which are likely to become darker and more apparent in the future. There are a variety of chemical and laser light treatments available to help lighten these spots and make the skin tone more uniform, but many people with age spots choose to use more natural methods like apple cider vinegar to get the same results.

Apple cider vinegar can aid in the regeneration of damaged skin cells because of the potent antioxidants it contains in the form of vitamin C and beta carotene.

Besides repairing the skin's cells, ACV regenerates your skin cells and improves the appearance of old spots by regenerating the skin's surface.

Combine ½ cup of ACV with 1 cup of water to form a topical aid.

For 30 minutes, three times a day, use a towelette to connect with these places.

Many people have said that after just a few weeks of treatment, old parts of their bodies looked very different.

When you drink a typical ACV drink, your body can help regenerate skin cells and fight off free radicals.

In order to make a drink, you'll need to mix:

- 1 tablespoon of ACV
- A cup of water

Drink every day.

Eradicating Acne

Blemishes that appear on the face, neck, chest, back, and arms have long been a problem for acne patients. Prescription medications and over-the-counter remedies can be pricey, ineffective, or include harmful ingredients and additives, which is why they should be avoided whenever possible. Acne patients can use apple cider vinegar in a variety of ways to treat their condition safely, organically, and efficiently. There are four effective treatment approaches (such as soaking, tonic, topical treatment, or facial mask) that might be used with apple cider vinegar that are inexpensive, easy to use, and risk-free! It's a common belief that apple cider vinegar, when applied to the skin in the form of a soak, bath, face cleanser, or mask, will help ease the root causes of acne and prevent recurrences in the future. If you apply apple cider vinegar directly to your skin, it works in concert with your body's natural antioxidant defense system to:

- Maintain a normal pH level in your skin's top layer;
- Control your oil production to avoid clogging your pores
- Reduce inflammation at acne's source
- Improve the flow of blood through the skin to lessen the appearance of acne's redness and other side effects.

The following ingredients should be combined to make an ACV soak:

In a bathtub full of water, add 2-4 cups of ACV

Take a 30-minute bath.

A tonic can be made by combining the following:

- 1 cup of water
- 1 tablespoon of ACV

Drink every day.

Make a topical therapy by mixing:

- ½ cup of ACV
- ½ cup of water

Use it as often as your skin requires.

The following ingredients go into a facial mask:

- ½ mashed avocado
- ½ cup of ACV

Apply evenly on your face for 10minutes, then rinse with lukewarm water.

Treatment for Varicose Veins: What You Can Do

This condition is characterized by a group of bulging or discolored veins that might cause pain and discomfort, or they can simply be a visual nuisance. As a result of increased pressure and decreased circulation, varicose veins are most commonly found in people's legs, feet, and ankles. Tight-fitting clothing, standing or walking for long periods of time, and crossing one's legs when sitting are all risk factors for varicose veins. Varicose veins can be avoided by doing the following:

- wearing looser clothing
- improving your nutrition
- staying well-hydrated

- When you're sitting down, put your feet up so that you can rub and massage your weak limbs to relieve the stress on them.

Apple cider vinegar has also been found to be an effective treatment for varicose veins. It can help keep the legs, ankles, and feet healthy by eliminating toxins and dead cells from the affected areas while also helping to detoxify the blood. ACV has these beneficial properties because it improves blood flow.

To prepare a drink, simply blend the following ingredients in a blender:

- 1 cup of coconut milk
- 1 cup of strawberries (or kiwi or other tropical fruit)
- 1 tablespoon of ACV
- Ice (as needed)

Make a smoothie and drink it every day until you have the right consistency for you.

You'll need about ½ cup of water and ½ cup of apple cider vinegar to prepare a topical treatment.

Every time you use this mixture, soak a towel or washcloth in the mixture and apply it directly to the veins for around 20–30 minutes.

Using this localized treatment, you can reduce the inflammation in your skin and veins, as well as improve your overall blood flow.

How to Make Your Own Deodorant

There are a variety of things that might cause body odor, including perspiration, bacteria, and clothing that restricts or creases, enabling moisture to remain (like armpits), where bacteria can thrive. Numerous people aren't aware that store-bought deodorants contain chemicals that are immediately applied to the thin skin layer that covers lymph nodes and veins in the armpit. Deodorants and antiperspirants have a highway of veins and nodes that move blood. The blood absorbs the chemicals and additives and moves them around the body in the bloodstream.

People are choosing natural deodorants because they don't want to put their health at risk by using chemicals in their products, which can cause a variety of unwanted effects. Apple cider vinegar can be used as an efficient deodorant without causing harm to the user's health and can even help to improve it.

This is everything you'll need to make a DIY deodorant:

- 1 tablespoon of normal water
- 1 tablespoon of ACV

Using a cotton ball, apply the mixture on thr armpit or area of odor and let it dry.

It is absorbed into the bloodstream, where it kills germs that cause odors and infections. Assuring adequate nutrient delivery to all of the body's systems is one way it can support the body's daily operations.

To make a preventative drink, mix 1 cup of water with 1 tablespoon of apple cider vinegar.

Drinking it on a regular basis will provide you with health-promoting vitamins, minerals, and antioxidants that keep germs that cause bad breath from reproducing in your torso and on your skin.

Free Bonus

Download my **"Keto Cookbook with 60+ Keto Recipes For Your Personal Enjoyment"** Ebook For **FREE!**

The **Keto Diet Cookbook** is a collection of **60+ delicious recipes** that are easy and fun to make in the comfort of your own home. It gives you the exact *recipes that you can use to prepare meals for any moment of the day, breakfast, lunch, dinner, and even dessert.*

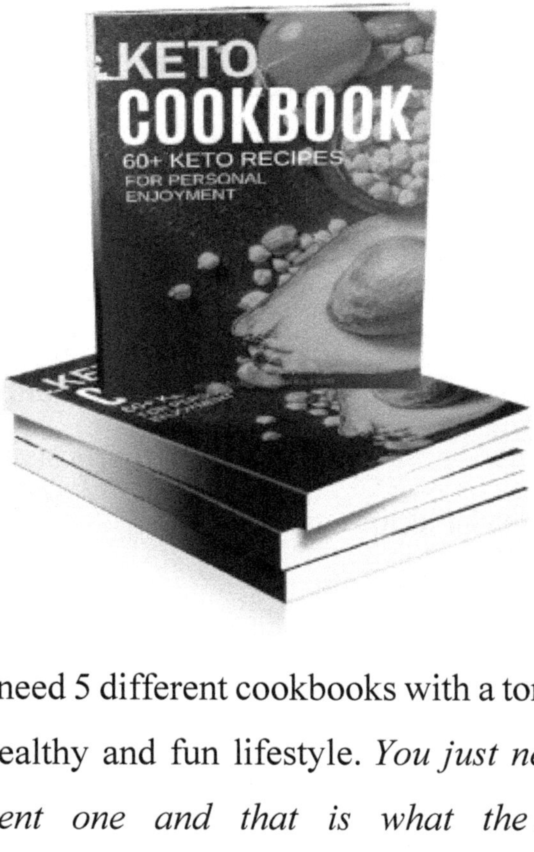

You don't need 5 different cookbooks with a ton of recipes to live a healthy and fun lifestyle. *You just need a good and efficient one and that is what the* ***Keto Diet***

Cookbook *is.*

Click the URL below to **Download the Book For FREE**, and also Subscribe for Free books, giveaways, and new releases by me. **https://mayobook.com/drmichelle**

Feedback

I'd like to express my gratitude to you for choosing to read this book, Thank you. I hope you got what you wanted from it. Your feedback as to whether I succeeded or not is greatly appreciated, as I went to great lengths to make it as helpful as possible.

I would be grateful if you could write me a review on the product detail page about how this book has helped you. Your review means a lot to me, as I would love to hear about your successes. Nothing makes me happier than knowing that my work has aided someone in achieving their goals and progressing in life; which would likewise motivate me to improve and serve you better, and also encourage other readers to get influenced positively by my work. Your feedback means so much to me, and I will never take it for granted.

However, if there is something you would love to tell me as to improve on my work, it is possible that you are not impressed enough, or you have a suggestion, errors, recommendation, or criticism for us to improve on; we are profoundly sorry for your experience (remember, we are human, we are not perfect, and we are constantly striving to improve).

Rather than leaving your displeasure feedback on the retail product page of this book, please send your feedback, suggestion, or complaint to us via E-mail to **"michelle@mayobook.com"** so that action can be taken quickly to ensure necessary correction, improvement, and implementation for the better reading experience.

I'm honored that you've read this book and that you enjoy it. I strive to provide you with the best reading experience possible.

Thank you, have a wonderful day!

About The Author

I help people to eat healthy food and live healthier lives. I have been a registered dietitian since 2005. In the past decade, I have helped hundreds of people to improve their health and wellbeing through nutrition. I am a licensed dietitian in the state of California and a member of the American Dietetic Association. I have been working in the wellness industry for over 10 years, and I have worked with people who have type 2 diabetes, high blood pressure, heart disease, weight gain, metabolic syndrome, and cancer. I understand that nutrition is key to good health, and I love helping people eat well.

My goal is to help people get healthy by providing them with a balanced diet, lifestyle changes, and support. My approach is holistic, which means that I look at diet as a whole, rather than focusing on one aspect.

I am a holistic nutritionist. I help people change their eating habits and lifestyles so they can achieve and maintain a healthy weight and a happy, energetic lifestyle. I teach people how to eat well, and I help people find the balance between healthy food and food that they love. I also work with people who have cancer, diabetes, and other chronic conditions to help them live healthier lives. I offer personalized nutrition counseling and healthy meal planning. I have a master's degree in nutrition and a doctorate in nutritional science. I am a registered dietitian in the state of California and a member of the American Dietetic Association. I believe in a healthy lifestyle, and I help people find the best path to get there.

Subscribe to my Newsletter to download my Free Book, and also be informed about my new releases, and giveaways here: https://mayobook.com/drmichelle

Connect with me on my Facebook Page here: https://fb.me/MichelleEllenGleen

My Books

Alkaline Diet: The Secret to Healthy Living with Alkaline Foods (Healthy Food Lifestyle)

The Alkaline Diet Cookbook: Your Guide to Eating More Alkaline Foods, and Less Acidic Foods For Healthy Living (Healthy Food Lifestyle)

Ketogenic Diet For Beginners: Your Complete Keto Guide and Cookbook with Low Carb, High-Fat Recipes For Living The Keto Lifestyle

Anti Inflammatory Diet Cookbook For Beginners: 3-Week Quick & Delicious Meal Plan with Easy Recipes to Heal The Immune Systems and Restore Overall Health

Apple Cider Vinegar: A Quick, Easy, and Affordable Guide to the Health Benefits, and Healing Power of Apple Cider Vinegar (ACV)

Apple Cider Vinegar: The Amazing Guide on The Uses of ACV For Numerous Health Conditions, and How to Make it from Home

Brain Cancer Awareness: How to Help Your Brain Fight Brain Cancer

Dr. Sebi Cookbook: Alkaline Diet Nutritional Guide with Sea moss, Medicinal Herbal Teas, Smoothies, Desserts, Mushroom, Salads, Soups & More, to Rejuvenate the Body with 100+ Recipes

Skin Tag Removal: How To Get Rid of Your Skin Tags in Simple Steps